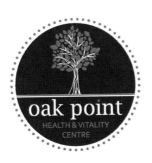

THE OAK POINT METHOD

THE A.R.T. OF
TREATING PAIN & CREATING
A SUCCESSFUL PRACTICE

BY DIMITRI BOULES
L.Ac, LMT, CPE, CPT

THE OAK POINT METHOD
The A.R.T. of Treating Pain & Creating a Successful Practice
By Dimitri Boules L.Ac, LMT, CPE, CPT

info@oakpointhealth.com
www.oakpointhealth.com

First edition
Published 2016
Edited by Mickey Z.
Designed by Eleni Louca
Photography:
Frank Lopis
Shutterstock- 18234784
Shutterstock- 18234739
Shutterstock- 76258783
Shutterstock- 117767344
Shutterstock- 39157972

ISBN-13: 978-0692600870
ISBN-10: 0692600876

Written in U.S.A

I'd like to dedicate this book to my wife Anna for always being there for me and supporting me, and to our awesome children.

ACKNOWLEDGMENTS

There are many people I'd like to thank but the first and most important person is my wife Anna. She's the reason I was introduced to Acupuncture and Oriental Medicine, she helped me study while in school, and she consistently pushes me to reach my full potential as a husband, father, and acupuncturist. I love you.

I'd also like to thank my teachers both in acupuncture school and those I had the pleasure to learn from via continuing education courses and books. I believe it says a lot about people when they are willing to share their knowledge so we can all improve and help as many patients as possible.

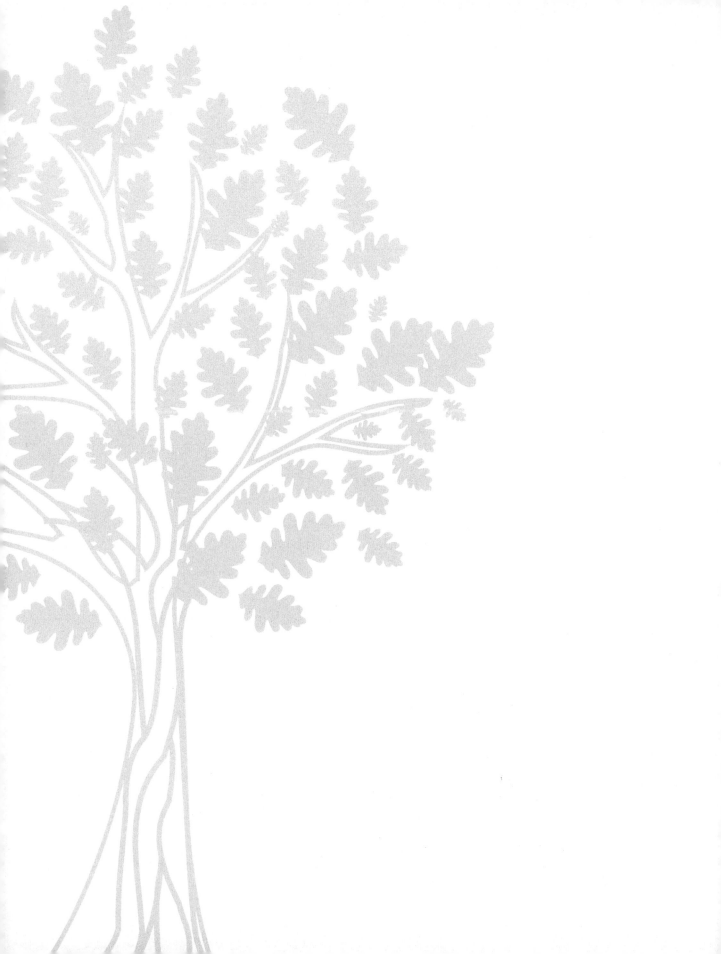

TABLE OF CONTENTS

Author's Introduction

Thank you for taking time to read *The Oak Point Method*. I'm confident you'll find the information contained herein to be both useful and innovative.

In my clinical work, by combining Oriental Medicine (acupuncture, tui-na, and other TCM modalities) with contemporary/medical acupuncture, I've helped patients with musculoskeletal conditions (MSK) achieve exceptional results. I'd now love to share my integrative approach with you.

My goal with *The Oak Point Method* is to offer a complete system along with the tools that will not only help more people but will also bring acupuncture further into mainstream awareness and acceptance—particularly in the field of neuromuscular skeletal medicine. What I'm proposing is a linking of the past (traditional acupuncture) with the present (modern acupuncture and functional assessment) to create a new path towards a future that embraces an even more holistic and integrated vision of assessment and treatment.

Just as practitioners all throughout history have adapted their theories and treatments, today's TCM professionals must relentlessly strive to evolve our medicine. We must do so, however, without ever forgetting where we came from and the original ideas that informed us.

Consider this: Only 10% of visits to Western-trained doctors result in a referral to a complementary and alternative modality (CAM). We know how effective this form of natural medicine is, especially in the treatment of pain. Imagine a world in which such practitioners are confidently referring patients presenting with pain to integrative acupuncturists instead of reflexively writing prescriptions and suggesting surgery. That's the kind of world I want to live in and the goal I'm aiming for.

I am by no means a "Master Acupuncturist" and I have not been guided by a "Guru." What I've done is seek out as many sources as possible—books, courses, etc.—outside of my college curriculum in order to stay perpetually in a state of learning. This approach has allowed me to put new and old ideas into practice and discover what's most effective for each of my patients.

My academic acupuncture program was run by Traditional Chinese Medicine (TCM) doctors from China and our curriculum emphasized treating internal medical conditions more than treating muscle or joint pain. Because my instructors emphasized Zang Fu theory—using herbal medicine more than any other modality, I knew how to work very effectively with patients who had gall stones, thyroid imbalances, emotional issues, digestive problems, sleeping disorders and other internal medical conditions. However, many or most of the patients coming to my clinic (and even the college clinic) needed treatment for muscular skeletal pain. It feels as if less than half of my education was focused on treating the conditions that lead most people to try acupuncture.

After working as a personal trainer and massage therapist, I had entered the acupuncture profession with the intention of focusing on MSK pain. Yet, due to the limits of my traditional acupuncture education, my results were average in that realm.

Many such patients, during my internship and private practice, would discharge themselves because they were not seeing fast enough results within the first couple of sessions or because they plateaued after weeks of treatment. For me, this was simply not acceptable and that's when my quest for better treatment options commenced.

In *The Oak Point Method*, my approach will be much more functional and structural while still incorporating Zang Fu and TCM theories. This method will be outlined in a blueprint pattern, enabling you to tailor treatments depending on the patients' constitutional diagnosis as well as functional assessment. By combining the two styles of acupuncture, you'll find that patients will attain quicker, longer lasting results and, in addition, many of their Zang Fu-related ailments will improve! Our patients at Oak Point are regularly and happily stunned by the rapid results they experience and, not surprisingly, have become a valuable source of referrals.

As health practitioners, we should not only be interested in treating the area of pain. We must also focus on treating the underlying physical dysfunction (which is usually an area away from the site of pain). Our patients are much more than their symptoms thus, our approach must be equally as holistic.

> "What I've done is seek out as many sources as possible -books, courses, etc.- outside of my college curriculum in order to stay perpetually in a state of learning."

CHAPTER ONE

MEET JOE

To follow is the story of one of my patients. Joe first came to our office after trying both a traditional acupuncturist and conventional therapy with a Western-trained practitioner.

Joe was an active 27-year-old male, working as a personal trainer. He was exercising daily, doing things like weight training, high intensity interval style cardio; followed a healthy diet; and played rugby on the weekends. He'd had an ACL reconstructive surgery ten years prior to our meeting and was experiencing knee pain that got worse after playing rugby or undergoing an intense workout.

After the pain persisted for a couple of weeks, Joe first revisited the exercises and stretches he'd done during post-surgery physical therapy (PT) a decade earlier. He also stopped all lower body weight training, such as squats and lunges.

After a few weeks, the pain did not decrease so he made an appointment with his primary care doctor. The MD asked him some general questions and—without assessing or even touching the knee—prescribed an anti-inflammatory

and wrote a prescription for physical therapy. While Joe opted not to take the medication, he did perform some prescribed exercises. However, a couple of weeks passed without any major improvements.

By way of context, please bear in mind this was a highly conditioned patient capable of squatting 325 pounds. Weakness in the muscles around the knee were obviously not an issue. After eight sessions of exercises and stretches that he deemed "too simple," Joe felt no difference and ended up discharging himself.

Frustrated and still experiencing pain, Joe recalled social media posts he'd seen about professional athletes like Kobe Bryant receiving acupuncture to treat injuries and speed up recovery. So, he scheduled an appointment with a TCM-trained acupuncturist. (It's not my intention to bad mouth this particular acupuncturist but rather I feel it's essential to highlight the differences in how MSK conditions are treated.)

This acupuncturist did an evaluation, palpated his knee, and told him that his kidneys were weak, adding that Joe "should avoid the cold weather" (even though it was the dead of winter in New York City) and "stop eating shellfish for a few weeks." After that, the practitioner proceeded to needle local points around the knee and after the needles were removed, he burned some Moxa on what sounded like Heding.

Joe continued with acupuncture treatments for the recommended eight sessions, noticing only a temporary reduction in pain. However, after a workout, the pain would intensify again. He remembers wondering if acupuncture was something he'd have to do for the rest of your life because it could only offer temporary relief.

Disappointed, the "kidney deficient" patient discharged himself yet again and began to accept the possibility that he'd have to live with the pain from now on. After all, osteoarthritis and knee pain after an ACL surgery is very common.

A few weeks later, an unexpected breakthrough occurred. Joe was working with a client with chronic shoulder pain. He hadn't seen this particular client for a while so of course, he asked how his shoulder was feeling.

"It feels great," the client replied. "I went to an acupuncturist a few weeks ago and got some treatments. My shoulder is great after four sessions with him. I think we should start trying some overhead shoulder presses now."

During the workout, Joe continued asking his client about the acupuncturist he went to and learned that after just one needle, his client's shoulder felt much stronger. The acupuncturist, he was told, explained everything and laid out a clear plan to treat a shoulder issue that months of conventional therapy and self rehab did not address.

> "Go for a consultation, Joe's client urged. "It's free. You have nothing to lose."

"Go for a consultation," Joe's client urged. "It's free. You have nothing to lose. I'll give you the number before I leave."

Fast-forwarding a few days later, Joe was in our office. During the consultation, he expressed his frustration and I began to feel he didn't think we could help him. It seemed he didn't even really want to be there. He already tried acupuncture and, to him, it didn't work.

This is when I articulated how our approach was different than that of a traditional acupuncturist, urging him to at least try one session. If he didn't notice a difference after the first treatment, I'd offer no pressure for him to return. I made it crystal clear I didn't want to waste his time or money.

What happened, you wonder? Well, in the ensuing chapters, I will go over the treatment approach I took with Joe. For now, let's just say he was pain-free after just five treatments and still comes in once a month for "tune ups" while regularly referring patients to our office.

Chapter Two

Traditional Acupuncture

(Benefits and weaknesses of our medicine)

I believe Oriental Medicine may be more effective than Western Medicine in treating many chronic and acute conditions. I'm sure plenty of you reading this book agree and have directly witnessed this reality in one way or another. That said, I still think there's something lacking in Oriental Medicine when it comes to treating mechanical dysfunction of the MSK system. As I've said before, it's not enough to treat the area of pain effectively. It's extremely important, if not more important, to treat the area of dysfunction.

During acupuncture school, if a patient came in with knee pain, we did generalized "knee treatments" and added some points based on Zang Fu principles. On rare occasions, stim was used or secondary modalities such as Gua sha or Moxa but the treatment was almost always just a whole bunch of points around the knee. One or two points might have varied depending if it were Damp Bi, Hot Bi etc. but the overall points were always the same.

This basic approach was used for wherever pain occurred— shoulder, back, wrist, ankle, elbow, it didn't matter! Very quickly, I realized such a method was less than ideal and the

lack of long lasting results only reinforced my frustration. My classmates and I began to lose confidence in such an imprecise treatment plan that only addressed the area of pain.

Some of the many benefits of Oriental Medicine when treating MSK pain:

🌳 Distinguishes different types of pain syndromes. For example, Cold Damp Bi, Heat Bi, Wind Bi, etc. This allows the acupuncturist to tailor their treatment specific to what is affecting the channels.

🌳 Many times, pain is due to an internal organ/Zang Fu imbalance. By asking the "10 questions," looking at the tongue, and feeling the pulse, Oriental Medicine practitioners can zero in on which organ is out of balance and thus may be contributing to the pain a patient is experiencing.

🌳 We have many tools other the acupuncture needles to treat with. Cupping, Moxa, Gua sha, Tui-Na, Herbal Medicine, and Nutrition can be used in conjunction with acupuncture to address the issue from different angles. If pain is due to trauma and the internal organs are not the cause of the issue, strengthening the patient's overall body function will enhance the healing process.

The single glaring weakness of Oriental Medicine in treating MSK pain, in my opinion:

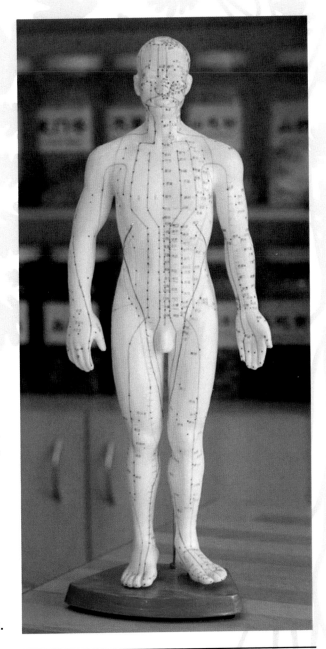

🌳 Not assessing and treating the mechanical dysfunction(s) that contribute to faulty movement patterns which, in turn, create a perfect scenario for acute injury, chronic abnormal wear and tear, or may even prevent an injury from fully healing.

To give you an idea of how drastically my methods have changed since acupuncture school, let's say there is a patient that was obviously in a great deal of pain and I only had one needle, I would use it to treat the area of dysfunction rather then the area of pain. By doing so, I assist the body to move optimally, improve distribution of forces, eliminate motor inhibition, and improve function which, in turn, will take pressure off the injured area and speed up the healing process. This is not to say that treating only the area of dysfunction is enough but, in my humble opinion, it's the most important part of our treatment plan.

CHAPTER THREE

MODERN MEDICAL ACUPUNCTURE

NOTE

"Using modern neurology and surface anatomy along with OM theory will set you apart from other practitioners."

Upon opening my own clinic, I discovered that 80% of my clientele came to me for treatment of muscle and joint pain. Therefore, we began seeking out many courses that specifically focused on these areas.

One such course was "Neurofunctional Acupuncture," taught by Dan Wunderlich LAcu, a practitioner who taught Medical Acupuncture to the U.S. military. In the short description of the course, Wunderlich highlighted the many doctors who took his course and came away extremely impressed with the results they were getting using this modality that was totally new to them. What fully sold me was when Wunderlich talked about the immediate results his patients were experiencing. I knew right then and there that I wanted to take his course. I simply could not wait to learn the techniques I felt were missing from my acupuncture education.

Wunderlich's approach, both fairly simple and extremely effective, involves three steps:

1 Needle the affected spinal segments that innervate the area of pain as well as the sympathetic vascular reflex.

2 Needle the homologous microsystem sites (I use the ear microsystem).

3 Needle the peripheral/local inputs (local trigger points, motor points, joint capsules, and nerve trucks).

For example, if a patient comes in with knee pain, the areas needled would be:

Spinal segmental and vascular reflex points: Huato Jia Ji points T10-L4

Microsystem: Ear knee point

Local/peripheral points: the motor point for the vastus medialis, the motor point for the tibialis anterior and the joint capsule of the knee.

Within one weekend of completing the neurofunctional courses, I was using these techniques in my clinic. Without telling my existing patients about the new approach I learned in this awesome acupuncture seminar, I simply applied the techniques and waited to see their reaction.

One by one, they definitely took notice and were extremely happy with the results. After just one session, I saw a drastic improvement in range of motion, decreased soreness, and most importantly, pain reduced and in many cases: eliminated. This not only pleased and motivated me, it got my patients feeling excited and hopeful. After years of unsuccessful treatment experiences elsewhere, they were seeing and feeling results at Oak Point!

Benefits of Modern Medical Acupuncture

- Uses modern anatomy of muscles and nerves
- Is a system that can easily be replicated

Weaknesses of Modern Medical Acupuncture

- Does not take into consideration the patient's constitution
- Does not differentiate patterns of pain (such as Cold Bi, Damp Bi, etc.)
- Does not address internal imbalances of the Zang Fu organs

One can see that when we combine the traditional form of medicine with modern acupuncture, we are addressing dysfunction, area of pain, and internal imbalances to treat the whole person rather then just the injury. This is why we blend the modern knowledge of anatomy with the traditional understanding of Oriental Medicine (OM) to yield faster and long lasting results.

CHAPTER FOUR

BEFORE WE TREAT, WE NEED TO ASSESS FOR DYSFUNCTION

NOTE

"He who goes to the site of pain without treating the dysfunction is lost."

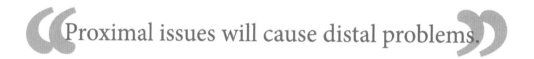

"Proximal issues will cause distal problems."

What is dysfunction?

Dysfunction is when certain muscles around the shoulder and hip girdle are inhibited and prevent the joints and muscles above and below those areas to move optimally. Proximal issues will cause distal problems. I often give the analogy of a car and its wheel alignment. If the car's alignment is off, there will be way too much abnormal wear and tear on the tires causing them to wear down quicker then usual. Just by changing the tires, the "dysfunction" is not addressed causing an ongoing issue. However, if the wheel alignment is addressed, the forces will be distributed evenly and the tires won't need to constantly be changed. An example of how this could present on our body is when we have a re-occurent elbow issue. Inhibition of the serratus anterior muscle will cause the shoulder and upper extremity to move abnormally resulting in dysfunctional movement patterns and elbow pain. We can treat the elbow every time without having long lasting results. It is like changing the tires. The root cause of the problem also needs to be addressed (in the above case the serratus anterior weakness) in order to get rid of the dysfunction and eliminate the problem once and for all.

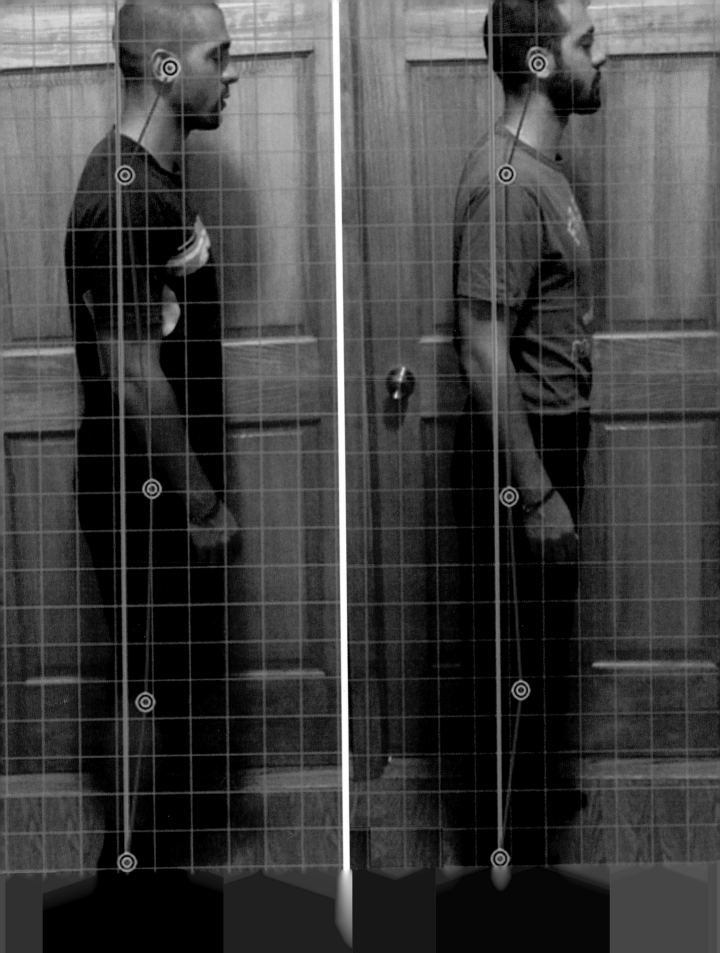

CHAPTER FIVE

THE EXSTORE ASSESSMENT SYSTEM

Often, the path towards excellent results commences in research. For example, I stumbled upon a series of short YouTube videos of a doctor going through a functional assessment which, at first, appeared too simple to be effective. Still, something piqued my curiosity so I dug deeper.

My digging led me to videos of Dr. Anthony J. Lombardi, creator of the Exstore Assessment System, going through an examination and treatment of a high performance athlete. It took no more than seven minutes to complete—from beginning to end. I could not believe how quick, precise, and effective this assessment/treatment was. As a skeptic, I had to find out more.

Short videos and brief explanations are not enough for me. I find it hard to settle for the bare minimum. After getting a brief glimpse, I wanted to know the rationale, theory, research; I wanted to learn the full assessment system so I ordered Lombardi's DVD/booklet combo.

While I would, of course, recommend going to exstore.ca and ordering the material for yourself, I will offer a brief explanation of how the Exstore System addresses the dysfunction underlying a patient's immediate symptoms.

Reminder: By identifying and treating the dysfunction, we will address the root cause of the problem, thus ensuring that the patient has a speedy recovery and help prevent the injury from reoccurring in the future.

Initial Session

After the patient has detailed their primary complaint, I clearly explain that I won't be treating solely the area of pain. I involve the patient in the process by making certain they understand that an area of dysfunction—despite not being located near the area of pain—is most likely contributing to the problem.

I feel it's important for them to know that treating only the area of pain may result in temporary relief but in order to heal faster with long lasting results, we must address the mechanical dysfunction. From my experience, patients understand and appreciate that I'm going above and beyond to address their issues.

Upper Body Exstore Assessment

For any neck or upper extremity condition (wrist, elbow, or shoulder), I perform the following assessment because, if the shoulder girdle is not functioning properly, it will create dysfunctional movement. This, in turn, will cause the joints below and above the shoulder to move abnormally. All this adds up to the perfect recipe for chronic pain or injury.

These are the muscles to be checked during the upper body assessment:

- Serratus anterior
- External rotators of shoulder
- Internal rotators of shoulder
- Supraspinatus
- Anterior deltoid
- Middle deltoid
- Posterior deltoid

If any of these muscles are found to be weak or inhibited, we must restore the dysfunction using electro-acupuncture. Below are the assessment factors to consider and points to use.

Please bear in mind: We always assess the non-affected side first in order to compare the results with those of the affected part of the body. After identifying the inhibited and/or weak muscle(s), we needle the appropriate motor point and stim them, using a handheld device for 30 seconds (we use the Pointer Plus II).

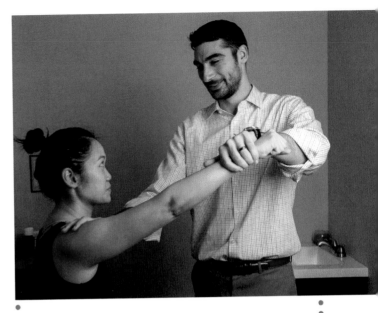

Serratus Anterior Assessment:

With the patient seated on the treatment table, have them flex the shoulder about 135 degrees while keeping their arm straight. At the wrist, the examiner should push down as the patient resists. Note any differences in strength between arms.

NOTE

Dr. Lombardi, of course, goes into ROM and other aspects of the assessment but these factors fall outside the scope of this book. If you're interested in learning the full assessment, again, I encourage you to order the packet and DVD.

Point to Treat:

Position the patient in side-lying and stand behind them. Move the lat muscle out of the way by grabbing and lifting it to expose the serratus anterior.

Needle in line with the nipple or about four cun inferior to the mid-axillary line.
Needle perpendicular to the tissue towards you.

Be extra cautious to not needle into the lungs. Stimulate the point with the Pointer Plus II for 30 sec to a few minutes. This will cause the muscle to contract and relax.

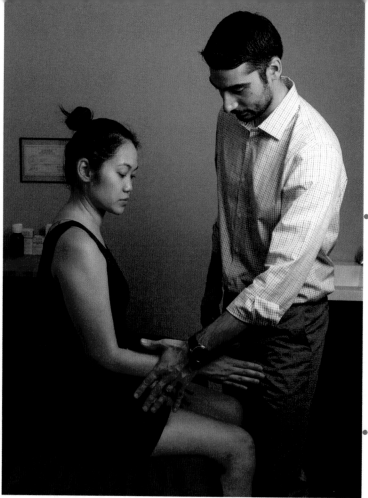

External Rotators Assessment: With the patient seated, have them bend their elbow to 90 degrees—with the elbow below the shoulder at all times. Ask the patient to rotate the bent arm outwards.

Points to Treat:

The two muscles responsible for external rotation of the shoulder are the infraspinatus and teres minor. Both muscles are part of the rotator cuff—a common site for injury.

If a patient has motor inhibition and weakness with external rotation, I typically needle both the infraspinatus and teres minor as they work together in order to perform the movement.

Point for Infraspinatus: Find SI12 and the inferior angle of the scapula and bisect it.

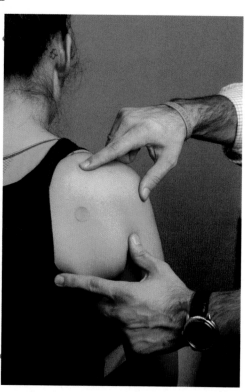

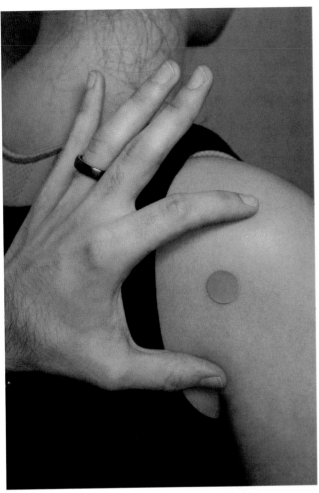

Point for the Teres Minor:
Find SI10 and SI9 and then bisect them. I refer to this point as SI9.5.

Internal Rotator Assessment:
With the patient seated, have them bend their elbow to 90 degrees—with the elbow below the shoulder at all times. Ask the patient to rotate the bent arm inwards.

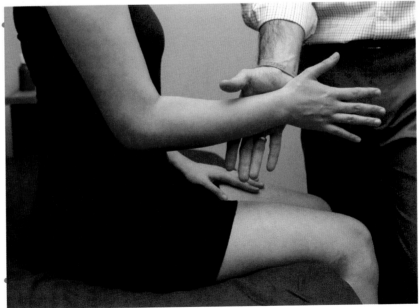

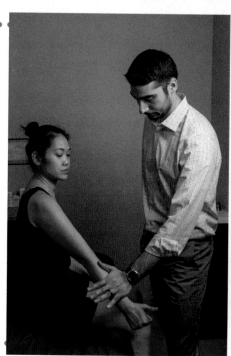

Point to Treat:

To access the subscapularis muscle, have the patient lying in supine with their arm abducted and their palm under their head as if they were resting.

Grasping the scapula gently, push the tissue with your thumb toward the lung to create some space.

Needle lateral to your thumb to avoid a pneumothorax and direct the needle posterior medially until you hit the sub scapular fossa.

I usually pull back slightly to ensure I'm only affecting the muscle and not the bone.

Supraspinatus Assessment:

With the patient seated, have them extend their elbow while the arm is in a 45 degree angle with the thumb up. The examiner should push down at the wrist level while they resist. Repeat with thumb down.

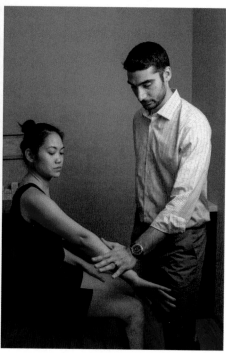

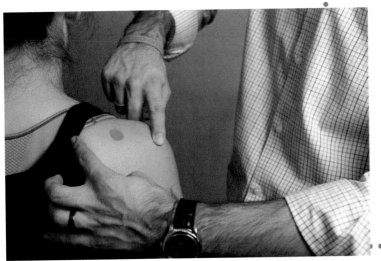

Point to Treat:

The supraspinatus motor point is located in the traditional SI12 point. I usually use a 1.5cun needle because it has to reach a motor point deep below the more superficial muscles (e.g. traps).

Needling should be perpendicular to the supraspinus fossa to avoid puncturing the lung.

Anterior Deltoid Assessment:

Have the patient flex their arm to 90 degree angle to their torso. Push down around the elbow as they resist.

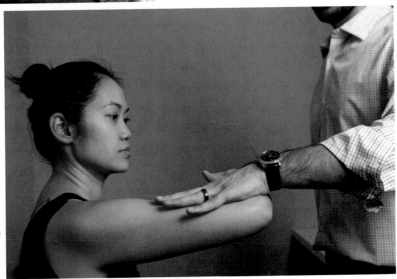

Point to Treat:

The anterior deltoid motor point is located midway between the anterior axillary fold and A/C joint.

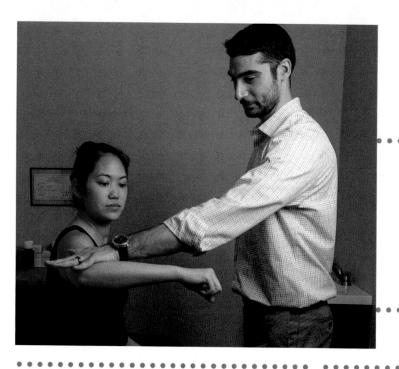

Middle Deltoid Assessment:

Have the patient abduct their elbow to 90 degrees. Push down around the elbow as they resist.

Point to Treat:

The mid-deltoid motor point is located 2.5cun inferior to SJ15 and one cun anteriorly.

Posterior Deltoid Assessment:

Have the patient adduct their elbow to 90 degrees. Pull the elbow anteriorly while the patient resists.

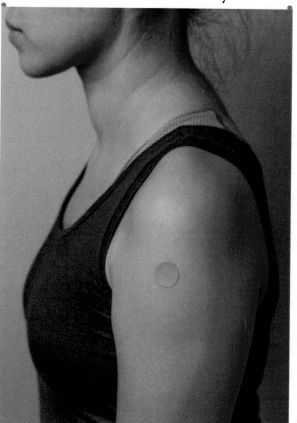

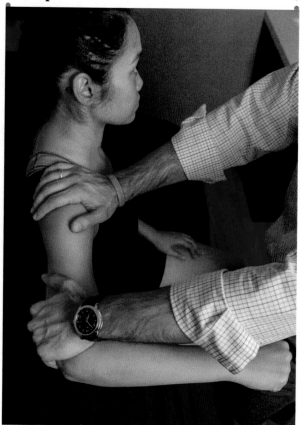

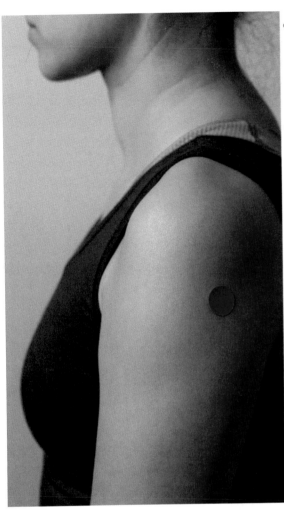

Point to Treat:
The posterior deltoid motor point is located 2.5 cun inferior to SJ14 and one cun posteriorly.

Lower Body

For lower body issues such as low back pain, hip, knee, or ankle injuries, I performed the Exstore Assessment for the same reason as mentioned above. Issues in the hip girdle will create dysfunctional movement patterns in the lower back and lower extremity.

These are the muscles to be checked during the lower body assessment:

- Obliques
- Hip flexor complex x2
- TFL
- Glute medius
- Glute minimus
- Glute maximus
- Adductors

Obliques Assessment:
Have the patient stand with feet about hip-width apart and arms extended in front of them. The examiner pushes the arms towards one side while the patient resists. Repeat for the other side.

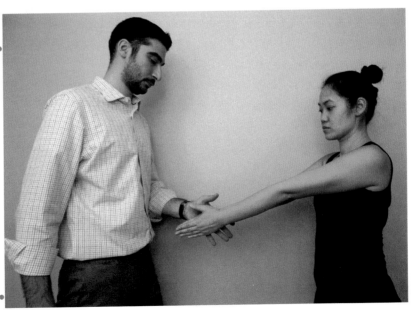

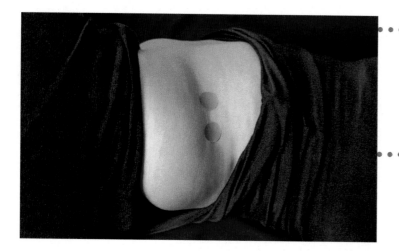

Point to Treat:

GBL26 on the weak/inhibited side. Motor point of the oblique muscles.

Hip Flexors (A) Assessment:

Have the patient lie supine and with their hip and knee both flexed to 90 degrees. Push the knee towards the foot end of the table while they resist.

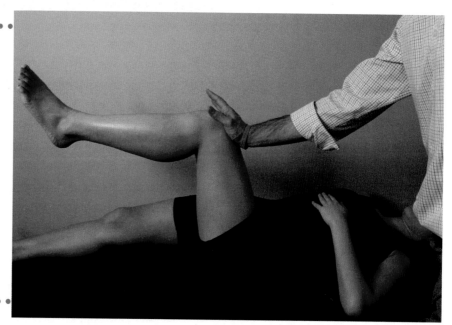

After the Exstore Assessment

After performing the Exstore Assessment, I needle the motor points of the inhibited muscles and then stimulate the needles with a pointer plus device to elicit a twitch response for 20-30 seconds on a frequency of 2-10 hertz—always making certain the patient is comfortable and the technique is painless. By painlessly stimulating the motor points, we help re-set the muscle and restore any motor inhibition.

Once that process is completed, I re-examine the previously weak muscle to ensure that it is firing properly before moving on to treat the area of pain. After the needles are removed, we perform Gua sha on the inhibited muscles to break down any scar tissue formation and reduce soreness.

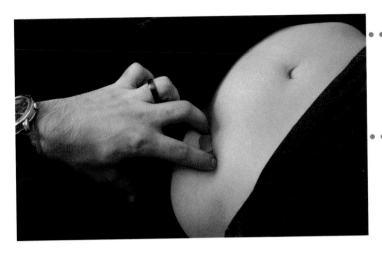

Point to Treat:
GBL28 thread towards the iliacus muscle. Motor point of the iliacus.

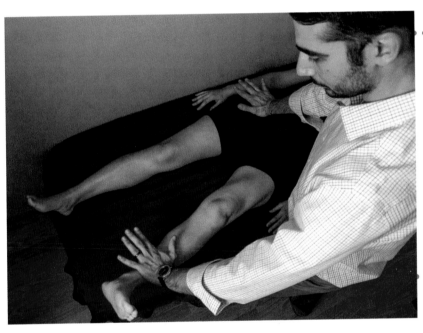

Hip Flexor (B) Assessment:
With the patient in supine, ask them to straighten the leg and lift it few inches off the table. Grasp the ankle and push it down towards the table.

NOTE

When muscles are chronically inhibited, scar tissues tends to develop which impedes the muscle's function. This is why we follow up with Gua sha after we restore the motor tissue.

TFL Assessment:

While the patient is in supine, internally rotate their lower leg and bring them in abduction. Have them resist adduction.

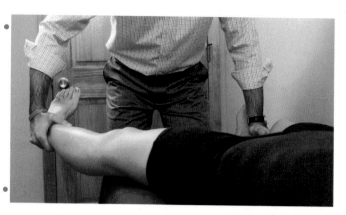

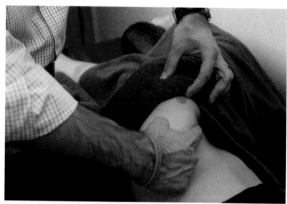

Point to Treat:

GBL29. Motor point of the TFL.

Glute Medius Assessment:

Same position as TFL but keep the lower leg in neutral. Patient should resist adduction.

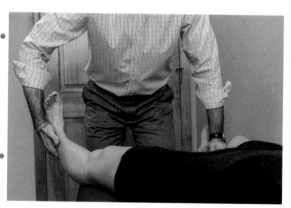

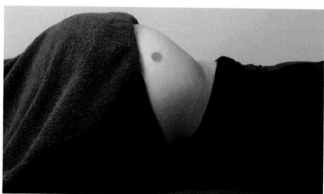

Point to Treat:

Five cun superior to the grater trochanter and one cun posterior. Motor point of the Glute Medius.

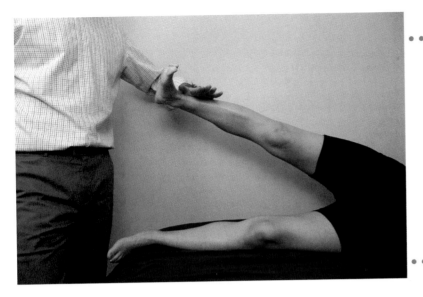

Glute Minimus Assessment:

The patient is in side lying with their leg in abduction. Grasp the ankle and push downward towards the table while the patient resists.

Point to Treat:

Halfway between the greater trochanter and the high point of the iliac crest is the motor point of the Glute Minimus.

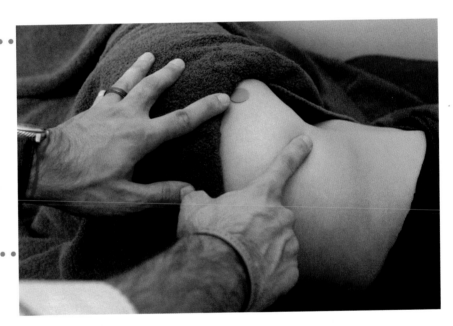

NOTE

If you would like to be part of our Facebook group and share your success stories and experiences using The Oak Point Method, email us a request to be added to our private group.

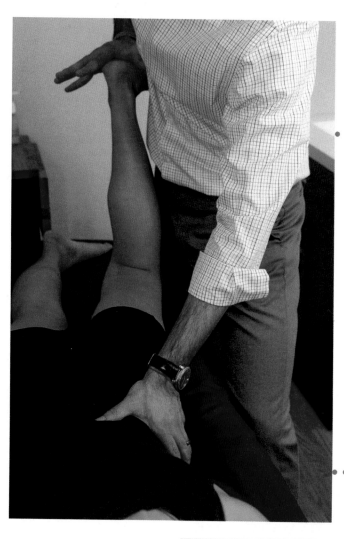

Glute Max Assessment:

Have the patient lying prone. Bend their knee to 90 degrees and ask them to raise their thigh off the table. The practitioner should grasp the foot and push downwards toward the table while the patient resists.

Point to Treat:

The motor point of the Glute Max is located 6cun lateral to S4 and 1cun inferior.

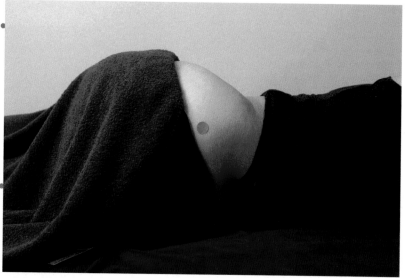

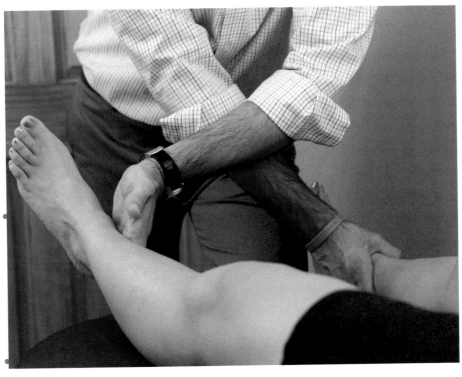

Adductors Assessment:
With the patient in supine, instruct them to resist abduction.

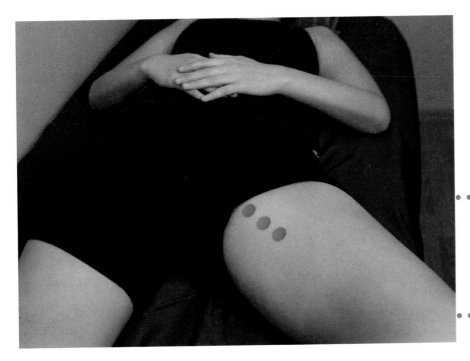

Point to Treat:
LV 10, 11 and or 12. Motor points of the Adductor group.

Chapter Six

Secondary Modalities

I rarely, if ever, perform only acupuncture on any patient as I've learned how secondary modalities enhance treatments and speed up healing. In addition, patients who've gone to other acupuncturists—practitioners who never did Tui Na or Gua sha on them—really appreciate that I do more then place some needles and leave them on the table for 30 minutes.

Secondary modalities not only enhance treatments but can also set you apart from other Western or Eastern medical practitioners. Your patients appreciate getting "more bang for their buck," even if they have to pay a little extra. To them, it's worth it because they see value in your service.

During the intake, I tell my patients that we'll be doing a lot of new things—especially in the beginning—and explain how each modality works and will help them with their condition. This increases both their curiosity about the treatments and their confidence in me as a practitioner.

When patients know you're going to use different modalities, it encourages them to come back for more treatments.

Here are the modalities we most commonly use:
- Tui Na
- Gua sha
- Cupping (sliding and static)
- Bone Setting/Joint Mobilization
- Moxa

NOTE

Of course, there are other OM techniques—7 Star needles, Ion Pumping Cords, bleeding, etc.—and if you use any of them in your practice, I encourage you to continue doing so. In my practice, I've found the above modalities to be not only most effective but also, the modalities our patients are most ready to accept and try.

At Oak Point, we usually perform one secondary modality on the painful area each time the patient comes in:

Session #1: Acupuncture and Tui Na massage. This will increase blood flow to the area, break down adhesions and trigger points, and relax the muscle tissues that may be injured or affected. Plus, most patients love getting a massage.

Session #2: Acupuncture and Gua sha (if applicable). This will increase blood flow to the injured area for up to seven hours, break down scar tissue, release fascial tension and muscle hypertonicity. Arya Neilson, PhD, conducted research on the biomechanisms of Gua sha and found that it increases profusion to the tissues up to 400% for the first 7 minutes.

Session #3: Acupuncture and Cupping (if applicable). We always do sliding cupping with some massage oil over the affected areas followed by static cupping, leaving the cups on for about 10 minutes. Beforehand, I explain to the patient that cupping is like a massage but instead of pushing their tissues down and compressing the area more, we are going to pull up and separate the tissues. This will flush out any waste products that have accumulated in the tight muscles and get fresh oxygen and blood to the area in order to facilitate healing.

Session #4: Acupuncture and Bone Setting/Joint Mobilization (if applicable and trained). In this session, I do some Tui Na on the affected areas before starting the Bone Setting/Joint Mobilization. To me, it makes more sense to relax the surrounding soft tissue in order for the Bone Set to stick and realign both soft and hard tissue.

Moxa is something we may also perform during the fourth session. We usually use it on joints like the ankle, knee, wrist, and lower back area if indicated. Moxa is great for arthritic conditions due to Cold, Damp, or a combination of the two.

NOTE

Even with good ventilation, the smell of Moxa can linger and thus, we do not use it extensively in our office. However, we sell poll Moxa to our patients and instruct them in proper home usage. At Oak Point, we use an infrared heat lamp to apply heat on the affected tissues instead of moxa.

After the fourth session, we usually use Tui Na and Bone Setting during every ensuing treatment and when appropriate, we will return to modalities like Cupping or Gua sha.

CHAPTER SEVEN

AUTHOR'S NOTES

Before we begin detailing the local treatments, I'd like to make a couple of clarifications to avoid any potential confusion.

1 Acupuncture Points.

In school, we learn the exact locations of each point on every meridian but, as Dr. Tan says in his lectures, acupuncture points are like the lines on a map. They are there to indicate where we are geographically but there are an infinite number of points between them! Thus, in my practice, I use the TCM locations but also palpate and needle the Ashi or tender point. If the actual BL58 location is not tender, I will feel around to discern the best location to needle.

2 Secondary Modalities.

Rather than repeat the same information for each body part, I will offer a key here:
First session: Tui Na
Second session: Gua sha
Third session: Cupping (sliding and static)
Fourth session: Bone Setting/Joint Mobilization and Tui Na

3 A.R.T.

To simplify your integration of the Oak Point Method, we have created an acronym (A.R.T.) for the three basic steps:

- Assess using the Exstore system
- Restore the motor inhibition
- Treat locally using TCM &
- Neurofunctional acupuncture apporach

ASSESS

RESTORE

TREAT

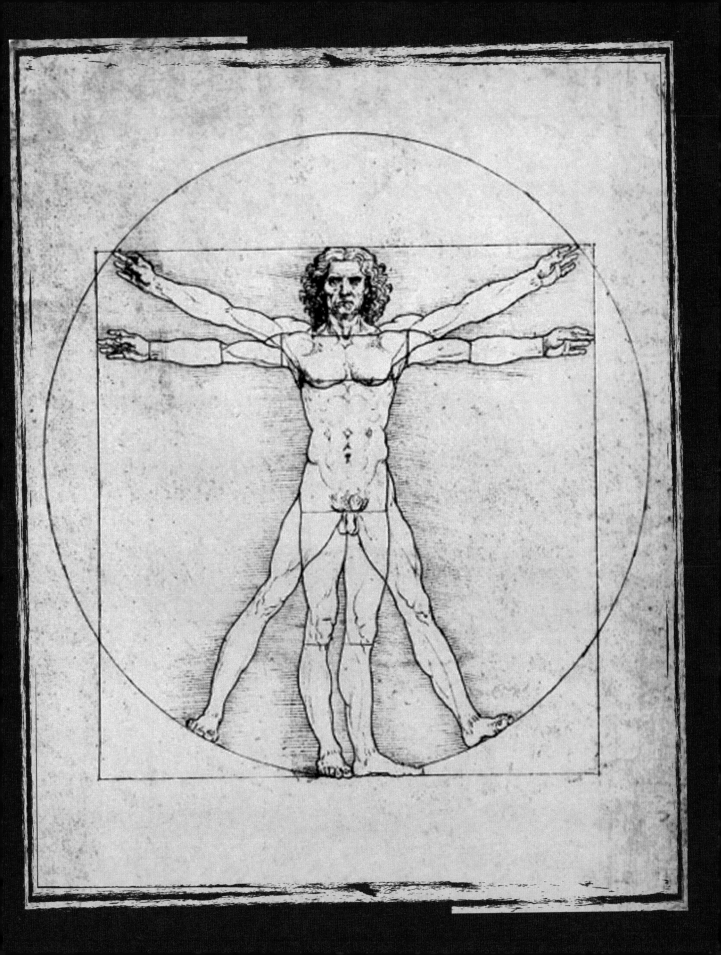

CHAPTER EIGHT

THE MOST COMMON CONDITIONS YOU WILL ENCOUNTER

NECK PAIN

I've found that the most common issue for patients with neck pain involves the levator scapulae and/or upper traps. Such patients, most often, present with upper cross syndrome which results in the head being far too forward and the posterior neck muscles overloaded with the task of trying to pull the head back into proper alignment. Eventually, of course, gravity wins and after chronic cervical strain, the upper traps, levator, and suboccipitals develop trigger points, adhesions, and spasms. It is also very common for patients that wear bags over their shoulder to develop neck issues since they are constantly contracting the upper traps and levator muscles to ensure that the straps do not slide off their shoulder. Even with a very light bag, we are subconsciously elevating our shoulder to keep the bag strap in place.

STEP 1: Assess for upper body dysfunction
STEP 2: Restore dysfunction
STEP 3: Treat locally

- **Cervical Huato Points**
  (even though Huato Jia Ji points are only in the thoracic and lumbar area, I will refer to these points as cervical Jia Ji points) of C3-6.
- **Traditional GBL21 point**
  (pain referring to the temporal area)
- **GBL21 posterior**
  (motor point/trigger point that refers pain to the sub occipital area)
- **GBL21 anterior**
  (pain referring towards the jaw)
- **DiJia**
  (levator scapulae motor point)
- **SI14 and SI15**
  (levator scapulae trigger points)

- Luo or distal points depending on what channel is involved and always picking the Ashi point
- Ear cervical spine
- **Points:** Depending on the TCM diagnosis.
- **Electro Stim:** I apply low frequency stim after I've used the pointer plus on the needles. Ideally, I'd like to provoke a muscle twitch from the levator and/or upper traps and focus the manipulation on 2 hertz for 10-15 minutes.
- **Heat Lamp:** Used after needles are set (if indicated)

STEP 4: Secondary Modalities

ANTERIOR SHOULDER PAIN

NOTE

"With anterior shoulder pain, look for postural distortion patterns that cause the shoulders to round forward. This puts the shoulder in a bad position and sets it up for injury. If upper cross syndrome is present, educate the patient on home stretches and exercises that will correct the muscle imbalance."

Anterior shoulder pain usually involves:

- **Suprasinatus tendon**
- **Biceps tendon**
- **Bursitis**
- **Ligament sprain**

This is a very common injury site, especially for those who regularly lift weights. Very often, patients experience discomfort after performing chest exercises like dips, wide bench press, and other movements that stress the structures listed above.

STEP 1: Assessment for the upper body dysfunction
STEP 2: Restore dysfunction
STEP 3: Treat locally

- **Huato Jia Ji points C4-T4** (C4-C5 are the spinal segments that supply the shoulder area and T1-T4 is the vascular reflex which will improve the profusion to the upper extremity.)
- **LI15**
- **Anterior Deltoid Motor point** Locate the AC joint and anterior axillary fold and bisect it.

- Ashi points on the area of pain
- Ear shoulder
- Depending on what channel is affected, pick LU or LI distal point below the elbow that is tender to the touch. Ex. LI4 or LU6
- TCM points depending on TCM diagnosis

- Electro Stim: Applied usually on the Anterior Deltoid as well as Ashi points in the front of the shoulder.
- Heat Lamp: (if indicated)

STEP 4: Secondary Modalities

POSTERIOR SHOULDER PAIN

NOTE

"Very common complaint from active individuals and athletes that perform Olympic style lifts such as cleans, snatches and deadlifts."

Posterior shoulder pain is usually caused by trigger points in the infraspinatus and/or teres minor muscles. When this common problem is addressed, our patients get more ROM and reduce the pain. It's common for those who perform Olympic-style weight lifting (deadlifts, cleans, etc.) to experience hypertonicity and trigger points on the external rotators of the shoulders.

STEP 1: Assessment for the upper body dysfunction

STEP 2: Restore dysfunction

STEP 3: Treat locally

- Huato Jia Ji points C-4 and C5 (because these spinal segments innervate the shoulder area)
- Huato Jia Ji points of T1-T4 area (the vascular reflex will increase blood flow to the upper extremity)
- SI10
- SI9
- SI9.5 is the point between SI10 and SI9 (motor point for the teres minor muscle)
- SI11 Ashi points. Usually I find the tight band on the infraspinatus in the area of SI11 and needle it with an inline pattern up to four needles.
- SI3 Ashi point (as a distal point for the posterior shoulder pain)

- **Teres Major Motor point**
  Locate the posterior axillary fold and move 1 cun superior and 1 cun medial.
- **Ear Shen Men and shoulder area.**
- **TCM points for the patients' constitutional diagnosis/type of Bi syndrome**

- **Electro Stim:** (usually applied on the most reactive points on the infraspinatus, SI10, and SI9.5)
- **Heat Lamp:** (if indicated)

STEP 4: Secondary Modalities

ELBOW PAIN

Before I started applying the Oak Point Method, medial and lateral epicondylitis was always something I found challenging to treat. The primary reason was because the dysfunction, which usually resides in the shoulder, was never addressed.

Medial Epicondylitis ("golfer's elbow")

STEP 1: Assessment for the upper body dysfunction
STEP 2: Restore dysfunction
STEP 3: Treat locally

- **Huato Jia Ji points C-7 and T1** (because these spinal segments enervate the medial elbow area)
- **Huato Jia Ji points of T1-T4 area** (the vascular reflex will increase blood flow to the upper extremity)
- **PC3**
- **HT3**

- **To find the Pronator Teres motor point, find the medial epicondyle and PC3. Draw a line from those two points moving distally and towards each other until they connect. The point where the two lines cross is the motor point of the pronator teres muscle.**
- **Ashi points near the elbow**
- **Ashi points on the flexor muscles of the wrist**
- **Ear Shen Men and elbow**
- **Depending on which meridian is involved, usually the HT, I would pick a distal Ashi point such as HT8-HT4**
- **TCM points for the patient's constitutional diagnosis**
- **Electro Stim:** usually applied on the motor point of pronator teres muscle, HT3 area, with maybe two more leads used on muscles in which the patient feels radiating pain.
- **Heat Lamp** (if applicable)

STEP 4: Secondary Modalities

NOTE

For the condition, I typically use Gua sha on the entire flexor muscle area—putting more focus on the medial epicondyle and common attachment of the flexors. Cupping the forearms can be difficult however, if you can get the cups to stay, it can be a good secondary modality.

Lateral Epicondylitis

A common condition for those with desk jobs or anyone who has to constantly perform movements with their hands, this condition is also known as "tennis elbow." While I have yet to encounter a tennis player with lateral epicondylitis, I've had plenty of secretaries, writers and mechanics come into our office with complaints about how this condition hampers their work and their lives.

STEP 1: Assessment for the upper body dysfunction
STEP 2: Restore dysfunction
STEP 3: Treat locally

- Huato Jia Ji points C6 (because the spinal segments enervate the medial elbow area)
- Huato Jia Ji points of T1-T4 area (the vascular reflex will increase blood flow to the upper extremity)
- LI11
- LI10
- LI9
- Locate the motor point, find the lateral epicondyle and LU5. Draw a line from those two points moving distally and towards each other until they connect. The point where the two lines cross is the motor point of the supinator muscle. (Motor point of the supinator muscle which has a common attachment site as most of the extensors of the wrist) Ashi points on the extensor muscles of the wrist
- Ear Shen Men and elbow
- Depending on which meridian is involved, usually the LI, I would pick a distal Ashi point such as LI4
- TCM points for the patient's constitutional diagnosis
- Electro Stim: usually applied on the motor point of supinator muscle, around LI10 area with two more leads used on muscles in which the patient feels radiating pain.
- Heat Lamp (if applicable)

STEP 4: Secondary Modalities
For the condition, I typically use Gua sha on the entire extensor muscle area—putting more focus on the lateral epicondyle and common attachment of the extensors. Cupping the forearms can be difficult however, if you can get the cups to stay, it can be a good secondary modality.

BICEPS STRAIN

While it's more common to see proximal injury to the long and short head of the biceps tendon, distal strain does occur and it's usually due to overloading the muscle doing something like biceps curls or trying to catch something heavy as it is falling.

STEP 1: Assessment for the upper body dysfunction

STEP 2: Restore dysfunction

STEP 3: Treat locally

🌳 **Huato Jia Ji Points C5-T4** (the spinal segments that supply shoulder area and T1-T4 area the vascular reflex which will increase blood flow to the upper extremity)

🌳 **LI15**

🌳 **LI14**

🌳 **Motor points of biceps brachii, #1 located 4 cun inferior from the anterior axillary fold and #2 5 cun distal to the anterior axillary fold and 1 cun medial.**

🌳 **Motor point of brachialis located 4-5 cun superior to LU5.**

🌳 **Depending on what meridian is affected, pick LU or LI distal point below the elbow that is tender to the touch. Ex. LI4 or LU6**

🌳 **Ear Shen men or biceps area**

🌳 **TCM points depending on TCM diagnosis**

🌳 **Electro Stim on the Motor Points of biceps brachii, brachioradialis and the distal portion of the attachment.**

🌳 **Heat Lamp**

STEP 4: Secondary Modalities

LOW BACK

Since many of our patients are gym goers and weekend warriors, it's not unusual to have visits from those who've tweaked their backs. More often than not, the problem stems from somewhere else, most commonly: weakness in TFL and glutes. By finding the source of the problem, we help speed up recovery and prevent re-injury.

STEP 1: Assessment for the lower body dysfunction

STEP 2: Restore dysfunction

STEP 3: Treat locally

🌳 **Huato Jia Ji points L3-L5** (because the spinal segments enervate the lower back)

🌳 **Huato Jia Ji points of T10-L1 area** (the vascular reflex will increase blood flow to the lower back as well as lower extremities)

🌳 **BL23-26**

🌳 **BL52**

"80% of the population will experience lower back pain at some point in their life. Learn how to treat it effectively and you will get a constant stream of referrals."

- Motor point of the QL located 4cun lateral to L2. Important to note here that the angle of the needle insertion should be oblique towards the lumbar vertebrae.
- Motor point of the glute medium muscle (when trigger points develop there, they could refer pain in the lumbar region)
- Ashi points on the lumbar region
- Ear Shen Men and lumbar
- Depending on which meridian is involved (usually the Bladder) I would pick a distal Ashi point such as BL58

- TCM points for the patients constitutional diagnosis
- Electro Stim: usually applied on the lumbar points at which the patient feels discomfort and the motor points of the glute medius (as well as trigger points)
- Heat Lamp

STEP 4: Secondary Modalities

HIP PAIN

While many patients come into our office with complaints of hip pain, it's rarely the result of an acute trauma/injury. More commonly, the culprit is chronic wear and tear which is often "diagnosed" as bursitis, arthritis, muscle spasm, muscle strain, labral tears, etc. With this in mind, as always, we should be interested in treating the area of dysfunction in order to restore proper function before addressing the area of pain.

STEP 1: Assessment for the lower body dysfunction
STEP 2: Restore dysfunction
STEP 3: Treat locally

- Huato Jia Ji points L1-L3 (because the spinal segments enervate the hip)
- Huato Jia Ji points of T10-L1 area (the vascular reflex which will increase blood flow to the hip as well as lower extremities)
- BL56
- GBL30
- GBL29
- Motor points of the glute medius, glute minimus, and glute maximus (muscles commonly involved in hip pain and dysfunction)
- Ashi points on the hip region
- Ear Shen Men and hip
- Depending on which meridian is involved (usually the Gall Bladder) I would pick a distal Ashi point such as GBL34 or GBL41

- TCM points for the patients constitutional diagnosis
- Electro Stim on the muscle motor points that the patient feels pain in.
- Heat Lamp (if applicable)

STEP 4: Secondary Modalities

KNEE PAIN

Under the knee cap

Do you remember Joe? If so, you'll recall he was presenting with anterior knee pain that worsened with activity. Joe had motor inhibition in the glute medius and TFL muscles on the affected side which caused abnormal wear and tear to his knee because the lower extremity was not functioning properly. Even though he'd been getting good "local" treatments, his previous practitioners only focused on his knee which was not really the problem.

There are many reasons why one may experience knee pain. In this section, we'll focus on knee pain felt under the knee cap—more likely a miniscus, ACL, PCL, arthritis type of issue—usually felt deep in the knee rather then on the sides.

STEP 1: Assessment for the lower body dysfunction
STEP 2: Restore dysfunction
STEP 3: Treat locally

- Huato Jia Ji points L3-L4 (because the spinal segments enervate the knee)
- Huato Jia Ji points of T10-L1 area (the vascular reflex will increase blood flow to the hip as well as lower extremities)
- ST36
- ST34
- SP9
- SP10
- Xiyan
- Motor point of the VMO muscle: slightly superior, lateral to SP10
- Ashi points on the knee region (ex. Heding)
- Ear Shen Men and Knee
- Depending on which meridian is involved (usually the Kidney and/or Liver), I would pick a distal Ashi point such as KD3 or LV3
- TCM points for the patient's constitutional diagnosis
- Electro Stim: on the VMO muscle connected to ST36. This will create a current going through the knee and area of pain. Then stimulate both XiYan points with high frequency.

- Heat Lamp (if applicable)

STEP 4: Secondary Modalities

LATERAL SIDE OF THE KNEE

Lateral knee pain is usually due to a tight IT Band. Many runners have this issue, especially those who start running long distances without adequate preparation. I almost always find dysfunction in the hip with this condition and thus use that as my starting point.

STEP 1: Assessment for the lower body dysfunction

STEP 2: Restore dysfunction

STEP 3: Treat locally

- Huato Jia Ji points L4-L5 (because the spinal segments enervate the knee)
- Huato Jia Ji points of T10-L1 area (the vascular reflex will increase blood flow to the hip as well as lower extremities)
- GBL33
- GBL34
- GBL31
- GBL32
- Motor point of the Vastus Lateralis muscle located 8 cun proximal to the superior lateral angle of the patella
- Ashi points on the IT Band. I usually do an in line technique with four needles about a cun apart
- Ear Shen Men and knee
- Usually the meridian involved is the Gall Bladder, thus points such as GBL41 or GBL 39 are used for distal points
- TCM points for the patient's constitutional diagnosis
- Electro Stim: focused on the Vastus Lateralis and IT Band.
- Heat Lamp (if applicable)

STEP 4: Secondary Modalities

NOTE

Cupping is a technique we use often with this condition—especially in the first treatment. Our goal is to create a little space in the lateral knee area as well as remove any stagnation that may be present. After the initial session, we perform Gua sha on the lateral knee to break down any scar tissue that may have built up between the IT band and Vastus Lateralis. After the third treatment, we usually perform Tui Na as well as Bone Setting for the lower spine, hip, and knee. These techniques help restore proper motion in the joints.

ANKLE PAIN

(acute sprain)

As acute ankle sprains are not unusual for athletes who train outdoors, it's not surprising that we see many patients with this complaint. Even thought Rest-Ice-Compression-Elevation (R.I.C.E.) is the most common choice of action for this ailment, I've attained far better results with a combination of acupuncture and Herbal Gao applications. The swelling, pain, and bruising typically reduces within 24 hours and thus, patients are able to add rehab exercises to strengthen the ankle joint faster and return to what they love doing in no time.

NOTE

Since acute ankle injuries are usually very painful and the joint is swollen and bruised, I typically just do acupuncture and send them home with herbal "ice" gao (more about that in the next chapter).

STEP 1: Assessment for the lower body dysfunction

STEP 2: Restore dysfunction

STEP 3: Treat locally

- Huato Jia Ji points L5-S1
- Huato Jia Ji points of T10-L1 area (the vascular reflex which will increase blood flow to the hip as well as lower extremities)
- BL60
- BL62
- GBL33
- Motor point of the tibialis posterior located 5cun superior to medial maliolus.
- GBL34': located 2 finger breaths inferior to the fibular head, motor point of the peroneal muscles
- Ear Shen Men and Ankle
- Usually the meridian involved is the Gall Bladder thus, include points such as GBL41 and GBL44 used for distal points.
- TCM points for the patient's constitutional diagnosis
- Electro Stim: usually applied on tibialis posterior and GBL34'. These muscles create a "stirrup" that supports the ankle. By stimulating these points, we strengthen the muscles that support and stabilize the ankle and are therefore most typically inhibited after an injury. This approach not only speeds up the healing process, it also increases the stability to prevent re-injury of the ankle. Also, I will connect one lead crossing the ankle

(ex GBL39 with GBL 41) to create a current running through the ankle instead of needling directly into a painful and swollen area. Since it is not recommended to needle directly into swollen, inflamed tissues, such crossing of the joint will reduce swelling and speed up healing.

🌳 Herbal: After the acupuncture treatment, an Herbal Gao is applied onto the ankle before we wrap it with an ACE bandage.

🌳 Ankle Pain (Subacute/Chronic)

Within 48 hours after the initial injury, patients treated with the method described above should notice reduced swelling and bruising. At this point, we will add a few extra points and techniques not indicated in the acute stage.

STEP 1: Assessment for the lower body dysfunction

STEP 2: Restore dysfunction

STEP 3: Treat locally

🌳 Huato Jia Ji points L5-S1 (because the spinal segments enervate the ankle)

🌳 Huato Jia Ji points of T10-L1 area (the vascular reflex which will increase blood flow to the hip as well as lower extremities)

🌳 BL60

🌳 BL62

🌳 GBL33

🌳 GBL40: Deep needling is required in order to reach the sinus tarsi. This requires a slight inversion of the ankle to "open" the joint for the needle to enter deeply

🌳 SP6 motor point on the tibialis posterior

🌳 GBL34': located 2 finger breaths inferior to the fibular head, motor point of the peroneal muscles

🌳 Ear Shen Men and Ankle

🌳 Usually the meridian involved is the Gall Bladder thus, include points such as GBL41 and GBL44 used for distal points.

🌳 TCM points for the patient's constitutional diagnosis

🌳 Electro Stim: We stimulate the areas we mentioned in the acute stage and add GBL40 using high frequency.

🌳 Heat Lamp (if applicable)

STEP 4: Secondary Modalities

NOTE

Tui-Na and bone setting are the go-to secondary modalities and we will give a Moxa poll to the patients to use at home.

NOTE

"Once you understand the Oak Point Method, you can apply A.R.T. to any muscular skeletal condition that comes through your clinic."

Chapter Nine

"That smelly magic stuff"

In the quest to expedite the healing process, I have some further suggestions to complement all the treatment approaches and ideas we just discussed. I'm referring to liniments, plasters, heat therapy, and more. By combining an integrated approach to acupuncture with the wisdom of Chinese Herbal Medicine, I've learned that patients get better and they keep coming back to buy "that smelly magic stuff."

Here's one example: A 76-year-old gymnast was practicing with his team, a week before a big show in Las Vegas, when he fell off a human pyramid and severely twisted his ankle. Fortunately, his son was a patient of mine and immediately called me. It was a Saturday and I was fully booked, however, as any dedicated practitioner would do, I asked them to come by after closing time so I could have a look.

The injured acrobat was carried into my office by his son and I could instantly see his left foot was swollen to twice its normal size. Honestly, it looked like something out of a cartoon. I was told he'd applied iced which, not surprisingly, caused more discomfort (see the end of this chapter for my "rant" on ice). I briefly explained how ice delays healing and that my goal was to take steps to help the body heal the injury, rather than just stopping the obvious, visual inflammation.

In this after hours treatment session, I performed the Oak Point Method acupuncture technique for ankles (see page 43) and then applied a San Huang Gao (herbal ice poultice) made by Zheng Gu Tui-Na and Kamwo. I told him again to eschew ice and instead, apply the poultice every 12 hours and loosely wrap his ankle with an ACE bandage.

Ankle sprains are one of the many specific cases for which I do not recommend rest but, of course, I'm also not suggesting a patient go for a run after they sprain or injure their ankle. In the case of the gymnast, I did recommend that, each morning, he move his ankle in whatever directions did not cause pain. For example, I told him to try writing out the entire alphabet three times with his toes. This exercise helps reduce scar tissue formation, strengthen inhibited muscles, and also pump excess fluid out to reduce swelling.

Not surprisingly, the patient was extremely nervous. Not only were we not doing

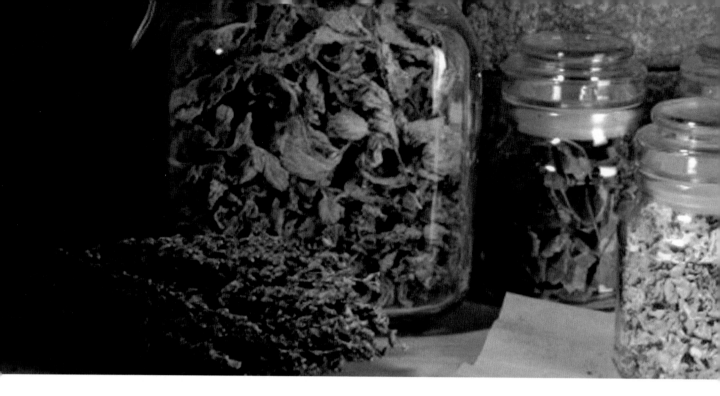

the "normal" route of icing, but he'd also never had acupuncture prior to this treatment. Since he'd heard such great feedback about our office from others at his gym, he decided to try. Before he left, I told him I'd meet him at his gym in two days (Monday, my day off) to re-evaluate him and perform another treatment since he had to travel on Thursday (less than a week after his initial acupuncture visit).

On Monday morning, I walked into the gym and there was the 76-year-old patient cleaning the place and presenting without a limp. I called out his name. He immediately waved to me, walked over briskly, and excitedly declared: "Look! The swelling went down and I have almost no pain!" Clearly, he was happy with the results and also relieved he was not going to disappoint his fellow teammates or miss the Las Vegas trip.

During our next encounter, I performed acupuncture on his ankle just to improve stability

and I added GBL 40 to stimulate directly in the ankle joint (something I did not do the first visit because of the excessive swelling and inflammation, see page 44). Lastly, after the acupuncture, I applied kinesiology tape to help stabilize the ankle.

The moral of this story? The Oak Point Method, combined with the Zheng Gu Tui-Na external products or any herbal product that is appropriate, helps the body to heal faster while intensifying the word-of-mouth buzz. Once again, everyone wins.

To follow, I'll offer a brief description of some topical and complementary treatments we use at Oak Point.

Liniments

Die Da Jiu (trauma liniment): For acute injuries, use within first 24 hours. Contains cooler herbs.

Zheng Gu Tui-Na (tendon liniment): For later

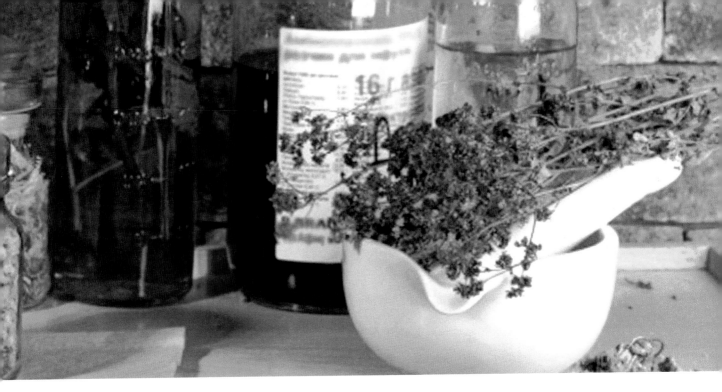

stage injuries, after the acute stage. Contains warmer herbs.

Plaster
San Huang Gao (also known as "herbal ice"): used for acute injuries or red, swollen areas of pain. Reduces inflammation and swelling while simultaneously removing stasis.

Herbal Medicine (oral)
Corydalis Natural Pain Relief Herb Pack (Non-addicting - Fast Acting by Pacific Herbs): Fifty percent pure Corydalis concentrated extract granules with seven additional herbs such as turmeric, known for improving circulation and decreasing inflammation. I've found that patients are more compliant with this herbal formula because of its relatively pleasant taste.

Heat Therapy
I recommend moist heat with many chronic and subacute injuries (joint or muscle) for 15-20 minutes—even when other health providers suggest ice. I've seen better results with moist heat both with my patients and myself.

Herbal Soaks
I typically use herbal soaks for any kind of foot or hand issue, e.g. arthritis, jammed fingers, ligament sprains, plantar fasciitis, and more. Depending on the injury, there are different soaks/herbs that the practitioner will prescribe. For example, if a patient sprains their ankle, we use a soak with cooling herbs instead of warming herbs to bring down the inflammation and swelling while at the same time removing stasis. On the other hand, when addressing a chronic injury that feels better with heat, we use a more warming soaks/herbs.

An herbal pharmacy will carry a variety of soaks (for Cold, Heat, Damp, etc.). They'll also have an all-purpose soak with different types of herbs and depending on what the patient needs, they can mix the specific herbs for their specific condition.

CHAPTER TEN

AS PROMISED, MY THOUGHTS ABOUT ICE AND RICE

Yes, I myself am guilty of using ice in the past. When I was working as a personal trainer and someone at the gym got hurt, we all ran for the ice. During my massage therapy education, ice was a major part of our treatments. I was taught that it helps reduce inflammation and stops swelling, and how we should inform our clients to R.I.C.E. (rest, ice, compression, elevation) after an acute injury. Even during my acupuncture program, ice was recommended and part of the patient's self care.

Much later, a full year after opening up our own clinic, we learned about the Oriental Medicine approach to acute injuries and, more specifically, their stance on using ice. I recall reading *The Tooth from the Tiger's Mouth* by Tom Bisio, a book in which it was explained why ice was not beneficial and what alternatives to use instead. It was truly eye-opening and since then, I've been advising patients to stay away from ice during the subacute or chronic stages and use more heat or herbal topical applications instead. I often quote Bisio's book: "ice is for dead people."

Whenever I treat a Western-trained health provider (including nurses, doctors, physical and occupational therapists), the topic of ice inevitably comes up. Of course, they repeat what they and I have been taught on the benefits of icing—especially for acute injuries. That's when I gently inform them that Gabe Mirkin, the M.D. who coined the term R.I.C.E., long ago admitted that he was incorrect because resting and icing actually delays healing. Let's break it down.

Ice: Let's say a person rolls their ankle while running. This means the tendons and ligaments in the area are inflamed and tight due to the injury, right? Well, let's consider what happens when we are out during a cold day: our muscles naturally tend to contract in order for our body to produce heat.
Combine these two concepts and you're left with this reality: A muscle is tight due to injury but we add ice to make the muscles even tighter.

This choice causes things to become static or—as described in Oreintal Medicine—qi and blood stagnation, which means energy, fresh blood, oxygen, and nutrients are not getting through the area of injury. If we're not able to get fresh nutrients to an injured area, how can we expect to speed up the healing process? Rather than stopping the inflammation by applying ice, we aim to help and assist the body in flushing out excess inflammation and increasing qi flow in the affected areas where there is an injury.

Rest: It's widely accepted that after an injury, our body lays down scar tissue in the process of repairing. Unfortunately, our body does a "sloppy" job and leaves the area looking and feeling different from its original form. This causes pain, maladaptation, faulty movement patterns, a decrease in ROM, and dysfunction.

By doing proper activities—and not resting—the scar tissue that forms is just the right amount and in the areas we truly need it. This is why immediately after knee replacement surgery, patients are encouraged to walk and start Physical Therapy to speed up recovery and return them to proper function a lot sooner than if they were to remain immobile. This type of information almost always inspires an open-minded Western practitioner to contemplate other perspectives and that's my cue to simply ask that they try our methods.

The worse case scenario is they don't see the results they want and go back to icing. Thankfully, I have "converted" all of them except one PT. He admits he felt better with moist heat but still says there's plenty of evidence that ice helps and thus, he still uses it with his patients. As you can see, challenging medical orthodoxy can be a full-time job!

NOTE

"Coaches have used my R.I.C.E. guidelines for decades, but now it appears that both ice and complete rest may delay healing instead of helping." Gabe Mirkin, MD, March 2014.

CHAPTER ELEVEN

THE OAK POINT BUSINESS MODEL

During acupuncture school, we were hit with the news that 80 percent of practitioners were not earning enough money to makes ends meet. Many acupuncturists, we were told, are supplementing their income through second jobs while others aren't practicing at all.

I never attended a business school or worked at a job that required me to "sell" my services—so I wondered if I'd end up as part of the 80 percent mentioned above. I also wondered why so many acupuncturists were unable to make a decent living.

These conversations had me believing that I'd have to go back to school after graduating from the Acupuncture program. I began looking into Naturopathy, Chiropractic, Physical Therapy, and even traditional medical school—not because I preferred these options or thought they were "better" than acupuncture but solely out of financial concerns. I still very much believed in the effectiveness of Acupuncture but began to imagine it was something I'd do on the side or as an extra service rather than a primary modality and my source of income would be derived elsewhere. Thank goodness

my wife encouraged me to stick with it and constantly boosted my confidence, assuring me we'd thrive.

Looking back at that time and those worries, I have new perspectives and would like to share my personal opinion on why so many acupuncturists are not making it:

1 We are not specializing

Acupuncture and Oriental Medicine, of course, treat the whole body and can very effectively treat many conditions. However, I believe each of us must find our niche. Seek out and discover what lights us up and leads to the best results. Specialization will create a buzz in your community and will make you stand out rather then blend in with everyone else. People will seek you out because patients like going to the best for their condition and not just another acupuncturist.

For example, due to my background in personal training and massage therapy, I have a good understanding of the MSK system and injuries. This is why I focused my practice on treating sports injuries, muscle and joint pain, as well as dysfunction. I've also focused all my continuing education on the treatment of those types of conditions from advanced Tui-Na, to contemporary acupuncture, corrective exercise and rehabilitation. I personally do not focus much on the treatment of emotional issues, digestive ailments or other internal medical conditions. For that, I have another acupuncturist working in my clinic that specializes in internal medical issues. Because of my specialization, I've become known for treating and helping patients with MSK conditions and they keep referring their friends and family to our practice.

So, find your niche and tirelessly seek out education within that realm. Become the go-to person for whatever you choose to specialize in—whether it be sports injuries, fertility, NAET, emotional issues, digestion, etc.

2 We are not comfortable asking for money
I certainly faced this issue when I first started. In fact, many of my classmates who were amazing practitioners simply did not feel comfortable asking for payments or recommending a series of sessions. I'm happy to report that I've addressed this issue in my own life but a recent experience taught me how common it is in our field.

When my wife gave birth to our son, we were both overworked and tired. My wife had her hands full taking care of a newborn and I was working more hours to cover for her while she was on maternity leave. For those who have children, you know sleep becomes a sweet, distant memory.

After a few months of having a jam-packed schedule at work and very little rest at home, I developed mid-back pain bilaterally, pain which caused discomfort while I was working. Usually, my wife would treat me but with our little guy keeping her occupied, I opted to seek out an acupuncturist in our area. Let's just say the experience was an eye-opener.

The practitioner arrived late to open the office, leaving me waiting outside in the cold for about 15 minutes. Knowing New York City traffic as I do, I gave her the benefit of the doubt and decided to look past this less-than-ideal first impression. It was what happened—or didn't happen—after the treatment session that alarmed me most.

On my way out, the acupuncturist asked how I felt. I explained that I felt better but still had discomfort. The provider did not ask me when I would come in next. She did not recommend a follow-up treatment. She didn't even mention having a plan to help me get rid of the problem altogether. All she said was: "Okay, well, give me a call if you would like to make another appointment."

Rather than explaining how many sessions I'd need and what it would cost, to me, her body language screamed: "I don't feel comfortable asking you to come back and having you pay me more money."

If you follow the Oak Point Method, it will increase your confidence as well as your results and hence make you more comfortable with asking for payments and suggesting long term treatment plans.

3   We often lack a plan

Without fail, every patient wants to know how many sessions it'll take before they see results and feel better. However, this is probably the hardest question for practitioners to answer because everyone responds differently to treatments. For example, an older patient with a chronic condition will probably need more treatments then a twenty year old who pulled their back a few days ago. With experience, we become better able to gauge how many sessions a given patient will need.

Sticking with the focus of this book, I'd like to share the treatment plan I suggest to patients with MSK pain and dysfunction during their first session:

Acute injuries: 4-6 treatments, twice a week
Chronic injuries: 8-10 treatments, twice a week
Maintenance: 1 and 2

After the last treatment (#6 or #10), we do a reevaluation to assess the results and the possible need for more sessions. If the patient has no pain, we move into the "Maintenance 1" phase: one session every two weeks for a total of six sessions. This approach helps wean them off the intense treatments and ensure that pain does not reoccur. In "Maintenance 2," we go with one session every four weeks for a total of six sessions. The focus continues to be on preventing a return of pain and keeping an eye on the old dysfunction or any new issues that might raise. An example of this is a patient with glute medius inhibition causing reoccurring lower back pain. During our monthly treatment, I will check for any dysfunction in the hip especially the glute medius muscle to ensure re-injury does not reoccur again.

As an incentive for patients to commit to the plan I recommend, I offer packages of 4, 6, 8 and 10 sessions and if they purchase all the recommended sessions on the spot, I also offer a slightly discounted rate.

For example:
4-pack: 5% off
6-pack: 10% off
8-pack: 15% off
10-pack: 20% off

Outcome #1: The bigger the package, the more they save. Customers like deals and saving money.

Outcome #2: This will increase your cash flow and fill up your schedule fairly quickly since we encourage the patient to schedule all their appointments for the weeks to come.

Let's see how this looks and plug in some numbers: You have three new patients on the schedule, each of whom can benefit from 10-pack. If your 10-pack costs $650 ($65 a session), instead of having an ending balance of $195 from those three patients (your regular fee per session), you'll have an ending balance for that day of $1,950.00 and you'll have 27 sessions already booked for the coming weeks.

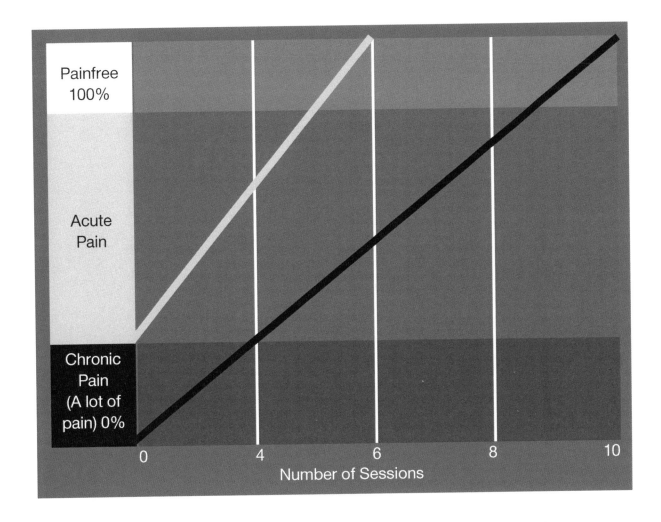

If you start off with just five new patients a week, each of purchasing a 10-pack, it comes out to $13,000 a month—from just five new patients per week! And this doesn't even include the possible sales of recommended herbal products. Not bad, huh?

The potential to make a living doing important work exists. We need an effective assessment system, a treatment protocol that makes sense and consistently gets results, and the confidence in our work and ourselves to get the patients to literally buy into the program.

As I said earlier, I once fell in the under-earn-ing trap but I've seen a great difference using the techniques and package business model described above.

Your goal might be just to make enough money to live an economically comfortable life. For me, using the system presented in this book gave me the ability for my practice to have good cash flow which allowed me to spend more time at home with my family while still making a good living doing what I love, wrote a book and take time off for long vacations. These are just some of the possibilities open to you when you embrace a system like the Oak Point Method.

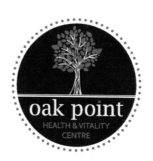

THE OAK POINT METHOD

THE A.R.T. OF
TREATING PAIN & CREATING
A SUCCESSFUL PRACTICE

BY DIMITRI BOULES
L.Ac, LMT, CPE, CPT

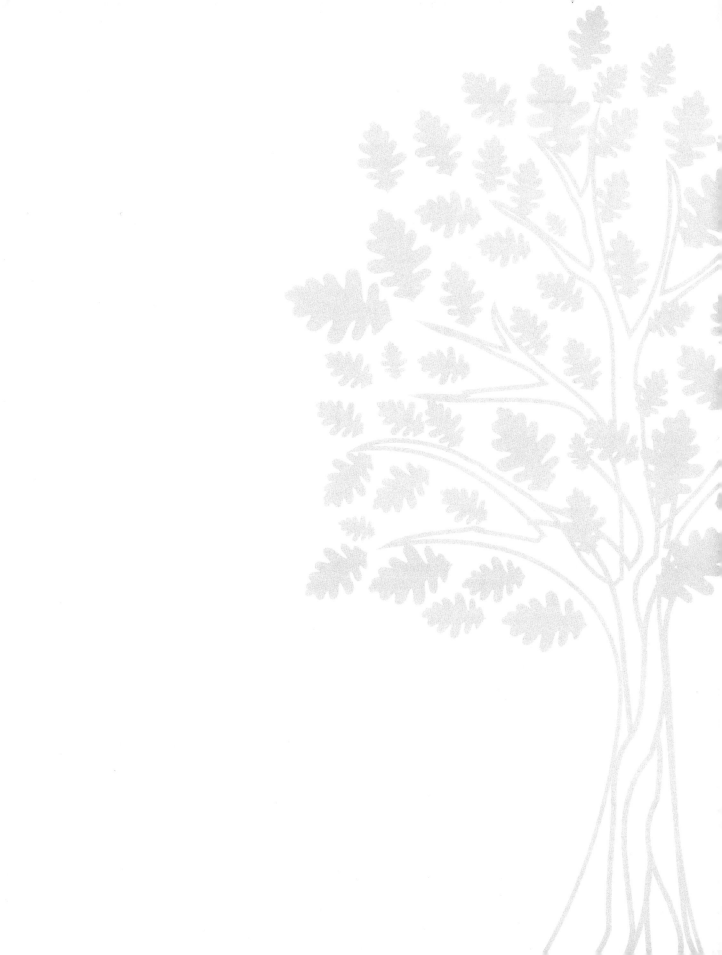

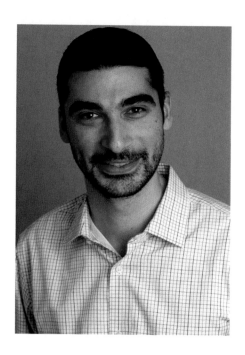

AUTHOR'S BIOGRAPHY

DIMITRI BOULES
L.Ac, LMT, CPE, CPT

As a New York State licensed acupuncturist and massage therapist, Dimitri takes a holistic approach with his patients—tailoring treatments to individual conditions and needs. He began working in the health field as an Astoria-based personal trainer in 2006 (National Academy of Sports Medicine certified). While he very much enjoyed helping people improve their health and fitness levels, he quickly recognized that the majority of his clients suffered from chronic pain or medical conditions. Many of them viewed pharmaceutical drugs and/or surgery as the only treatment options. Dimitri realized there were better alternatives and decided to continue his education.

He completed his degree in Massage Therapy and his Bachelors and Masters degrees in Acupuncture at New York College of Health Professions. Dimitri also completed a holistic health counseling program at the Institute for Integrative Nutrition as well as a certification in posture rehabilitation from the American Posture Institute. His education and learning has never stopped! Dimitri regularly attends seminars all around the world and voraciously reads the latest research in massage therapy, acupuncture, holistic health, and more.

Today, Dimitri is co-owner of Oak Point Health & Vitality Centre in Astoria, where he treats a wide range of conditions and concerns but specializes in neuromuscular skeletal problems, such as sports and orthopedic injuries, sciatica, lower back pain, etc. As the long list of happy Oak Point clients will attest, his blend of traditional and contemporary acupuncture, massage therapy, corrective exercises, and posture rehabilitation truly addresses the root cause of dysfunction and not just the symptoms.

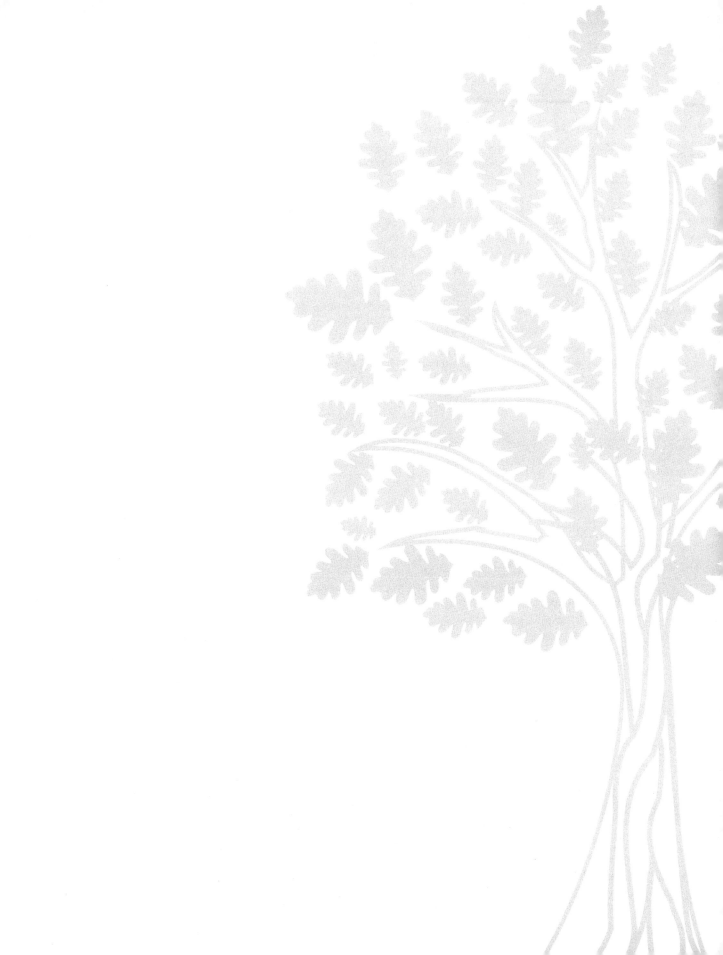

REFERENCES, RESOURCES, AND FURTHER READING

Books

Bauer, Matthew D. (2011). *Making Acupuncture Pay: Real-World Advice for Successful Private Practice*. Indianapolis, IN: Dog Ear Publishing, LLC. (cited on p. 56)

Bisio, Tom (2004). A Tooth from the Tiger's Mouth: How to Treat Your Injuries with Powerful Healing Secrets of the Great Chinese Warrior. New York: Fireside Books. (cited on p. 52)

Deadmen, Peter (2007). *A Manual of Acupuncture*. Journal of Chinese Medicine Publications; 2nd ed. Edition. (cited on pp. 38-48)

Lombardi, Anthony (2013). *Exstore Assessment System*. Hamilton, ONT: Hamilton Back Clinic PC. (cited on pp. 18-33)

Maciocia, Giovanni (2005). *The Foundations of Chinese Medicine: A Comprehensive Text for Acupuncturists and Herbalists*. London: Churchill Livingstone; 2nd edition. (cited on pp. 18-33)

Oleson, Terry (1996). *Auriculotherapy Manual: Chinese and Western Systems of Ear Acupuncture*. Health Care Alternatives; 2nd edition. (cited on pp. 38-48)

Tan, Richard Teh-Fu (2007). *Acupuncture 1,2,3*. Richard Tan. (cited on p. 36)

Xinnong, Cheng (2009). *Chinese Acupuncture and Moxibustion*. Beijing: Foreign Languages Press; 3rd Edition. (cited on pp. 38-48)

Seminars

"Motor Point Acupuncture." Instructor: Dr. Anthony Lombardi, 2015. Website: acupuncturemotorpoints.com (cited on pp.18-33 and pp. 38-48)

"Zheng Gu Tui Na." Instructor: Frank Butler, 2015. Website: zhenggutuina.com (cited on p.35)

"Neurofunctional Acupuncture." Instructor: Dan Wunderlich, 2013. Website: danwunderlich.com (cited on pp.16-17)

"National Academy of Sports Medicine," 2010. Website: nasm.org (cited on p. 38 and 44)

Articles

Mirkin, Gabe, MD. (2015). Why Ice Delays Recovery. http://www.drmirkin.com/fitness/why-ice-delays-recovery.html (cited on pp. 52-3)

Nielsen, Arya, PhD. (2012). The Science of Gua sha. Pacific College of Oriental Medicine Publication for the 24th Pacific Symposium. (cited on p. 35)

*Herbal recommendations mentioned on p. 51 sourced from:
Kamwoherbs.com
Pacherbs.com

Made in the USA
Middletown, DE
10 January 2020

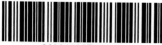